Stoner Quotes

Smashwords Edition License Notes

Publisher's Note

Speak On It: Celebrity Quotes About Marijuana

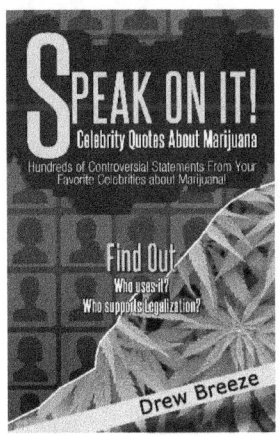

Hundreds of Celebrity Quotes about Marijuana, Cannabis, Weed, and Legalization. You will be surprised to learn who smokes marijuana and who supports legalization. Purchase this book and have instant access to the many controversial statements that have been made about marijuana! Check out these...

"Marijuana influenced negroes to look at white people in the eye, step on white men's shadows, and look at a white woman twice."

"I didn't live my life in the right way for politics, you know I f*cked too many chicks and did too many drugs, and that's the truth... I drank the bong water." ~George Clooney

If you smoke cigarettes or drink alcohol, you are not in a position to criticize weed smokers.

My friend prefers alcohol over weed. I prefer watching him clutching the toilet all night long, while I float in space.

Stoners have the best stories.

The best part about waking up is baking up.

A blunt a day keeps the drama away.

I don't do drugs. I set plants on fire and breathe.

Only pack what you can smoke.

Here's to the guy who looked at weed and was like, "Hey I wonder if we can smoke this shit!"

Cannabis: No violence, no hangovers, no problems.

Drunk drivers run stop signs. Stoners wait for them to turn green.

Smoking weed doesn't make me a bad person, just like going to church doesn't make you a good person.

Just saved tons on weed, by growing my own.

Be so blunt that they could smoke your truth.

Weed is not a drug. It's a plant. Therefore, I'm not a drug dealer, I'm a florist.

Never quit smoking weed. Nobody likes a quitter.

A doctor once told me, "Smoke weed every day."… Does Dr. Dre count?

I'm on a seaweed diet. I see weed, I smoke it.

Not sure if I smell weed or smell like weed.

The rules of weed do not work for pussy. If you can smell it across the room, it is not the good shit.

Not sure what's worse...waiting for the dealer when dry...or pizza when high.

Stoners live and stoners die. But in the end we all get high. So if in life you don't succeed, fuck that shit and smoke some weed.

Free your mind one puff at a time.

I finally found the pot at the end of the rainbow. But some idiot had already smoked it.

People call stoners lazy, but guess what assholes? The blunt doesn't pass itself.

A friend with weed is a friend indeed. But a friend who shares is a friend who cares.

In Colorado, marijuana got more votes than Obama.

I love smoking weed after a long day of smoking weed.

You can't buy happiness, but you can buy weed and that's pretty close.

Turn your blues into greens.

Stoner? I prefer the term "Cannabis Enthusiast"

If you smoke weed before an eating competition, does that mean you used performance enhancing drugs?

Marijuana is like sex, if I don't do it every day, I get a headache.

I like skinny girls but I'd never turn down a fatty.

Weed enhances life. Food tastes so much better. Music sounds so much cooler. Sex feels so much greater.

Fuck me, I'm stoned. If I get any higher, Google Earth will start paying me for images.

If you sell weed at an auction is it fair to sell it to the highest bidder.

I'm high on life. And weed. Mostly weed.

Marijuana is not a gateway drug. I don't know about you but I have never been smoking weed and said "Hey! Let's do some meth!"

I pledge to always smoke weed and never give a fuck.

Weed can turn strangers into best friends.

Mary Jane will always be my valentine.

The only thing weed kills is boredom.

Making cannabis illegal is saying nature made a mistake.

If marijuana makes you lazy, why are people worried that crime rates will go up upon legalization?

I don't have time to hate people who hate weed cause I'm too busy smoking with people who love weed.

If strippers are exotic dancers, aren't drug dealers exotic pharmacists?

You know what sucks about weed? Never enough weed.

Weed is legal in my house.

I smoke weed. You don't? Well I bet you're either an alcoholic or you take some sort of pills so let's keep our judgments to ourselves shall we?

A marijuana smoker is arrested every 37 seconds and you wonder why we're paranoid.

As part of a balanced breakfast on 4/20 don't forget to eat your weedies!

At 4:20 p.m. on April 20 millions of pot smokers around the world will observe 420, otherwise known as Weed Day, to mark the marijuana movement.

Be careful: Marijuana may cause intelligent thought, peacefulness, bliss, love, and the feeling of oneness with your surroundings.

Drunks blow through stop signs but stoners stop and wait for them to turn green.

Freedom doesn't exist as long as nature is illegal.

Fuck love and love weed.

God made weed. Man made beer. In God we should trust right?

Got busted with weed once and the cop asked me to give up my source. I said "Mother Earth."

Happy 420 Day.

High people understand other high people. They catch things that others don't.

How do you know you're a pothead? The last thing you studied for was a urine test.

I don't do drugs… I smoke weed.

I don't smoke weed to escape reality, I smoke weed to enjoy reality even more.

I got 99 problems and they all solved with Kush.

I only smoke blunts if they're rolled proper.

I'd rather have the munchies than a hangover!

I'd rather smoke weed and feel great all day, than drink alcohol and feel ill the next day.

I'm not addicted, I'm dedicated. So grab your bag and let's get medicated.

If laughter is the best medicine and marijuana makes you laugh. Is marijuana the best medicine?

If the ocean were weed and I was a duck, I'd swim to the bottom and smoke my way up. But the ocean ain't weed and I ain't a duck. So pass the bong and shut the fuck up.

If we all had a bong, then we'd all get along.

If weed is ever legalized, I can't wait to
see the commercials.

If you don't smoke, I don't know why.

Inhale the good shit, exhale the bad shit.

Inhale. Hold it. Exhale. Smile.

It's 420 somewhere!

It's a very strange thing when you make
nature illegal.

Let ya hair blow in the breeze. Roll some
bomb ass weed.

Marijuana Monday. Toke up Tuesday. Weed Wednesday. Faded Friday. Sour Diesel Saturday. Smoke Something Sunday.

People tell you to live above the influence, but when you're high you're above everything.

Real eyes realize real highs.

Reality is best experienced through red eyes.

Roll, roll, roll the joint,
Twist it at the end,
Grab a lighter and spark it up,
And share it with a friend!

Sex, drugs, and rock 'n' roll.
Speed, weed, and birth control.
Life's a bitch until we die,
So fuck this world, let's get high.

Sit back and take note while I take tokes
of that marijuana smoke.

Smoke good. Eat good. Live good.

Smoke it like you stole it!

Some people go to high school...others
go to school high.

Sorry for the bluntness, that's just how I
roll.

Stoners are chill.

Stress can pull you down, but weed can lift you right back up.

Struggle is the enemy. Weed is the remedy.

As the world turns, the kush burns.

There is a chemical in weed called "fuck it," and if you can just get that in your system, it can change your life.

To make marijuana against the law is like saying God made a mistake.

Weed: It's something to do, when there's nothing to do, that makes nothing to do, something to do.

Why drink and drive when you can
smoke and fly?

Yeah… I found the pot at the end of the
rainbow and I smoked it.

You can't complain when you've got
Mary Jane.

You never know how important your
lighter is until it's gone.

Being asked if I want to hit that is like
being asked if I want money.

Mary Jane is a woman you can trust.

When I'm sober, I do things. When I'm
high, I experience things.

Rolling all my problems into a blunt.

If you wake up, you gotta bake up...
That's the rule.

Weed might not be the answer, but it's a
damn good start.

You can't spell healthcare without THC.

When in doubt, bong it out.

It's okay to be fat, if you're a blunt.

THC stands for Toke Herbs Constantly.

I get high because I like the view.

Weed in, stress out.

Cereal cures two of the side effects of smoking weed. Hunger & Thirst.

They say money can't buy happiness. Wrong! I buy it in grams.

Whoever rolls it, sparks it.

Make sure you get your daily dose of your vitamins T, H, and C.

Weed is just nature's way of saying high.

Marijuana is responsible for causing 0 deaths a year. Worldwide, alcohol is responsible for causing 2.5 million deaths a year!

More weed, less stress.

Can't sleep? There's a weed for that.

When life gets tough and things get
tragic. Smoke a joint, it's fucking magic.

Mary Jane isn't a hoe. So don't just hit it
and quit it.

Cigarette smokers get free health care.
Weed smokers get one free phone call.

Newbies: Don't try to roll if you don't
know what you're doing, this isn't the
time to practice.

Inhale the good shit, exhale the bullshit.

According to the CDC, Tobacco use causes over 5 MILLION deaths a year.

Marijuana causes zero deaths and actually helps heal people.

If she can't roll, she's not the one.

You know you're high when everything you do feels like a mission.

Weed is a gateway drug to a better life.

Fire in the bowl, stress leaves my soul.

Under the influence, but above the ignorance.

There should be no drama in a smoking circle.

Do not disturb, when I'm with my herb.

Time for a date with Mary Jane.

My weed! My rules! and most importantly MY MUSIC!

God is perfect. Man is not. Man made liquor. God made pot.

Never quit smoking weed. Nobody likes a quitter.

This weed is too loud to hear your ignorance.

So many problems and one solution,
weed.

Marijuana is a gateway to happiness and
food. Not heroin and cocaine.

I wouldn't call weed a drug. I would call
it a miracle.

Cereal is one of the best things to eat
while high. The milk cures cotton mouth
and the cereal satisfies your hunger.

If she can roll, wife her.

Ash before you pass.

Bud so hard, motherfuckers wanna
grind me.

Hit bongs, not women.

Happiness can be found within a circle of friends lost in a cloud of weed smoke.

Bud Light? I'd rather Light Bud.

Smoking weed doesn't ruin your life. If you can't smoke weed and get shit done, blame yourself, not the weed.

Quality over Quantity.

Weed might not be for everyone, but everyone should try it.

Alcohol can destroy your liver. Tobacco can give you cancer. Weed can make you laugh.

Marijuana is a part of nature, so getting high is only natural.

If you climbed Mount Everest and lit up a blunt, you would be the highest person in existence.

Pills kill. Weed chills.

I'm high as heaven, but my eyes are low as hell.

I'd like to thank Mary Jane for being the realest woman out there.

Dankrupt means to be out of weed.

The most dangerous thing about weed is getting caught with it.

Go to class high, study high, take the test high, and get high grades.

Remember every time you don't clear a bong hoot that there's a non-high person out there wishing they had weed.

I smoke weed only on days with T's. Tuesday, Thursday, Today, and Tomorrow.

I only smoke weed on days that end in Y.

They call me alarm clock because my weed's so loud it wakes everyone in the morning.

I'm against animal abuse, but I hit white owls.

When you're high you don't just listen to the music, you start feeling the music.

You might be a stoner if your bong gets washed more than your dishes.

Don't start drama, smoke marijuana.

It's never okay to hit a women unless it's Mary Jane.

To my future kids: If I find weed in your room, I'm smoking that shit.

Please don't drink and drive, just park and spark!

So high I'm never coming down.

Smoking the best buds with your best buds.

If smoking weed is wrong, I don't want to be right.

Blunt wrap: $1.00. Weed: $20. Lighter: $1.99. Smoking, feeling great, and forgetting about my problems... Priceless!

I like to start my day on a high note.

Alcohol kills, weed chills.

A drunk will hit his wife. A stoner will hit his bong.

Some of my strongest friendships started
with a blunt.

I had a problem...but then I smoked
weed.

When life's a cunt, spark up a blunt.

Pass blunts, not rumors.

Always start your day on a high note.

Save your liver, blaze a swisher.

Eyes so low, mind so high.

Employers: A person should be judged by the quality of their work, NOT the quality of their piss.

Smoking weed is supposed to be a peaceful thing, so don't interrupt it with drama and bullshit.

Smoking the best, exhaling the stress.

You're a bowl pack away from a better day.

A blunt a day, keeps the doctor away.

Time to get fried on Friday.

Keep calm and get high.

Drama and weed don't mix.

I put my issues and my problems in my swishers.

Whoever said the best things in life are free, obviously grew their own weed.

When shit goes wrong, grab a bong.

They should make diet weed. It would be a strain of weed that doesn't give you the munchies and named "bud light."

I like my weed like I like my popcorn...with no seeds.

Stress can pull you down, but weed can lift you right back up.

Mary > Molly

I don't have a weed problem unless I run out of weed.

Legalize, Regulate, Educate, Medicate.

Smoking weed doesn't make you a bad person, just like going to church doesn't make you a good person.

Roll roll roll your joint,
Pass it down the line.
Take a toke, inhale the smoke, and
Blow your fucking mind.

If you're angry, hit Mary Jane. She doesn't mind.

A couple that smokes weed together, stays together.

Marijuana is not illegal because it's bad, it's bad because it's illegal.

If weed is a plant and plants are life...then wouldn't smoking weed be getting high on life?

Rosa Sparks - When you're so stoned that you refuse to get up.

Whoever invented the drug test is a real ass hole.

Roll it. Light it. Burn it down.

I keep it 420%

Wake up. Back up. Gotta get my cake up.

Don't kill the high because you're low.

God created the bees, the trees, and the marijuana seeds.

I had two bowls for breakfast. One was cereal.

My life is a constant battle between wanting to get high and not wanting to smoke all my weed.

When nothing goes right roll up and pass it to the left.

Walking around like my OG Kush don't stank.

Don't let the joint just burn while you're holding it. Puff, Puff, Pass.

I get by with a little help from my friends. I get high with a little help from my friends.

When life hands you lemons, make lemonade and smoke a blunt.

I'm so high I can vomit a comet.

Purple Haze got me in a daze.

Weed is bad, we should burn it.

I smoke so many trees I got splinters in my throat.

It's crazy how I stay so high and so down to earth.

Can't cope? Don't mope. There's hope. Smoke dope.

Comparing tobacco to weed is like comparing Hitler to Gandhi.

The only weed law we need is one protecting our right to it.

Find someone that loves weed as much as you do.

If you don't find time to smoke weed every day, I question your priorities.

Smoking weed is like having sex, it's a good idea anytime of the day.

Hoping all my problems blow away as I exhale.

The only time I breakdown is when I'm about to roll up.

Too high to care about the bullshit.

Keep calm and smoke weed.

Pot smokers are peace keepers.

Stay higher than the people trying to bring you down.

Maybe it's time to put down the cigarettes & stand up for weed.

Don't criticize it, legalize it.

Smoking weed will not ruin your life, but being caught with it can.

Kush cologne > Cig cologne

A tolerance break, is something I can't tolerate.

The people that think weed is bad, are the ones that need to research it.

Pass weed, not STDs.

My favorite side effects of smoking weed
are laughter & happiness.

Weed could save the world if we just let
it.

The only thing that is bad about
marijuana, is running out.

Weed is only a gateway drug to an open
mind.

Why don't I need Ritalin to focus,
Tylenol for headaches, or Advil for pain?
Marijuana is my medicine.

Explain to me why the average person doesn't question cigarettes being legal cancer and cannabis the cure being illegal.

Weed is only dangerous if you are caught with it.

Smoking weed. Side effects do not include: COPD, cancer, or death.

Weed is sunshine on a cloudy day.

I CAN'T HEAR YOU, my weed is too, loud!

Alcohol kills, marijuana chills.

The couple that blazes together stays together.

Smoke bongs & quote songs.

I'm not a morning person, but wake and bakes sure make it better.

Pass bongs, not judgment.

Smoking weed is like fitness, because even if you don't want to, you'll love the results.

No job, but always has money for weed.

Puff puff ash & pass.

Weed is less harmful than the consequences of being caught with it.

Weed is visine for your mind.

The smell of weed is better than the smell of cigarettes any day.

The dependence of weed is equal to the intoxication of caffeine.

Proof weed isn't addictive; Weed smokers want to smoke, tobacco smokers "HAVE" to smoke.

Marijuana is a killer, she'll murder your stress.

Weed can fix any bad mood.

Weed is a gift to help you live in the moment, so enjoy the present.

The only thing I can't do high, is pass a drug test.

Weed is my answer. Peace is your question.

When I decided weed over tobacco I knew I wasn't on the side of the law, but I know the law isn't on the side of my health.

If you never smoke weed you'll never know why people smoke weed.

Haters gonna hate, stoners gonna bake.

High Girls > Drunk Girls

You can be an educated intelligent
person and still smoke marijuana.

Smoke weed to feel good, not to fit in.

Don't act like an idiot when you're high.
You make the rest of us look bad.

I do my best thinking when I'm high.

I don't smoke weed to escape life. I
smoke weed to enhance it.

I don't have to smoke weed to have a
good time, but I always have a good time
when I smoke weed.

I don't get mad at people anymore, I get
high and say 'fuck em.'

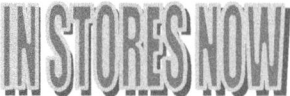

Speak On It: Celebrity Quotes About Marijuana

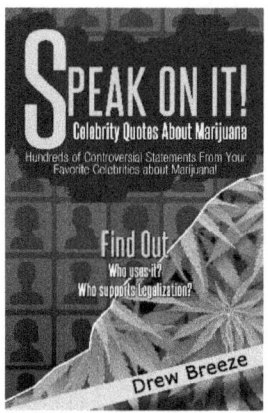

Hundreds of Celebrity Quotes about Marijuana, Cannabis, Weed, and Legalization. You will be surprised to learn who smokes marijuana and who supports legalization. Purchase this book and have instant access to the many controversial statements that have been made about marijuana! Check out these...

"Marijuana influenced negroes to look at white people in the eye, step on white men's shadows, and look at a white woman twice."

"I didn't live my life in the right way for politics, you know I f*cked too many chicks and did too many drugs, and that's the truth... I drank the bong water."~George Clooney

CONNECT WITH ME

FOLLOW ME ON TWITTER:
HTTPS://TWITTER.COM/DREWBREEZE420

FOLLOW ME ON INSTAGRAM:
HTTP://INSTAGRAM.COM/DREWBREEZE420

FAVORITE ME AT SMASHWORDS:
HTTPS://WWW.SMASHWORDS.COM/PROFILE/VIEW/DREWBREEZE420